Large Print Color by Numbers

Butterflies & Gardens
Coloring Book for Adults

ZenMaster Coloring Books

COLOR TEST PAGE

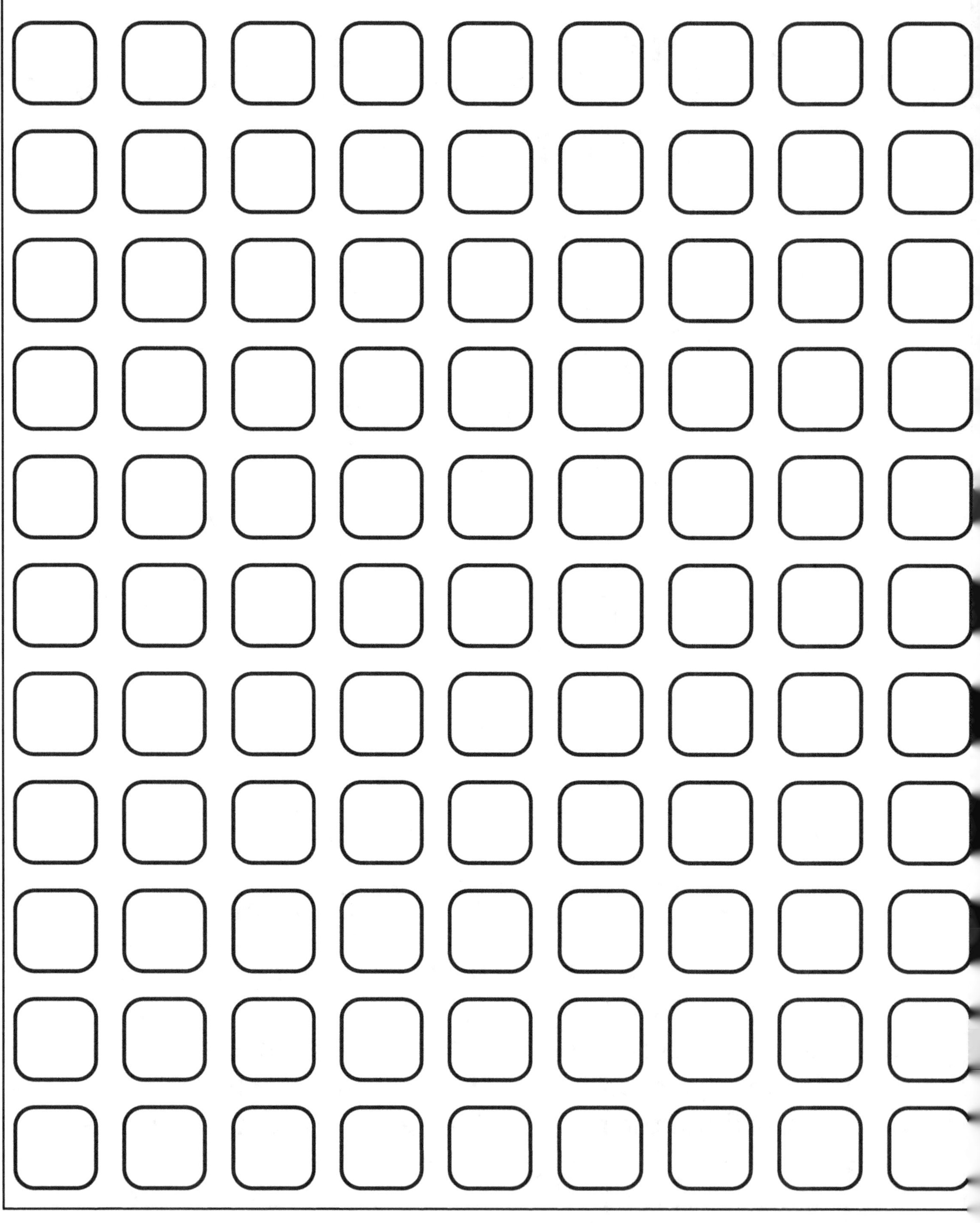

COLOR TEST PAGE

1. Yellow
2. Blue
3. Light Green
4. Orange
5. Magenta
6. Black
7. Dark Purple
8. Brown
9. Green
10. Dark Green
11. Pink
12. Red
13. Cyan
14. Purple

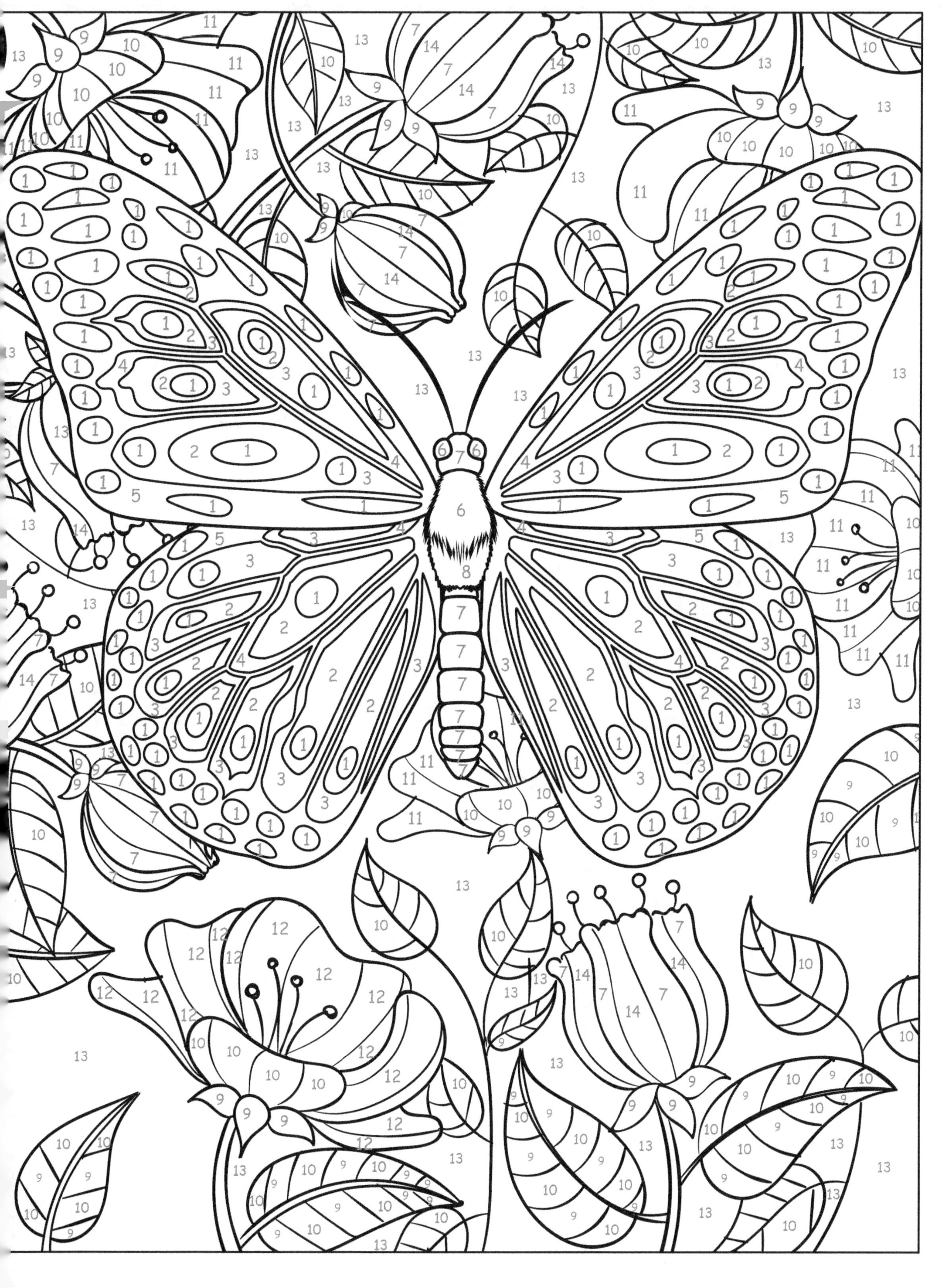

1. Yellow
2. Blue
3. Light Green
4. Orange
5. Magenta
6. Black
7. Dark Purple
8. Brown
9. Green
10. Dark Green
11. Pink
12. Red
13. Cyan
14. Purple

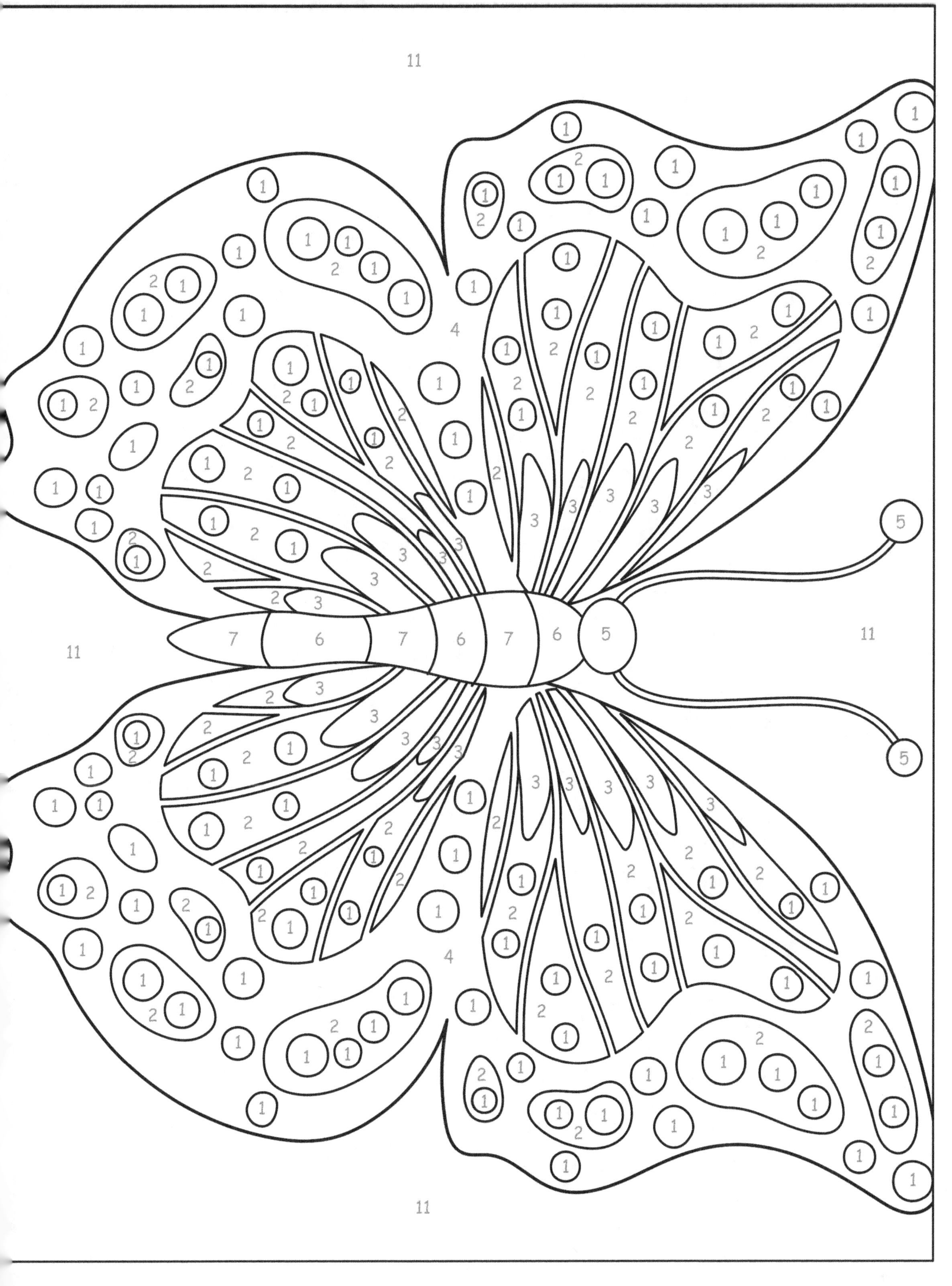

1. Yellow
2. Blue
3. Light Green
4. Orange
5. Magenta
6. Black
7. Dark Purple
8. Brown
9. Green
10. Dark Green
11. Pink
12. Red
13. Cyan
14. Purple

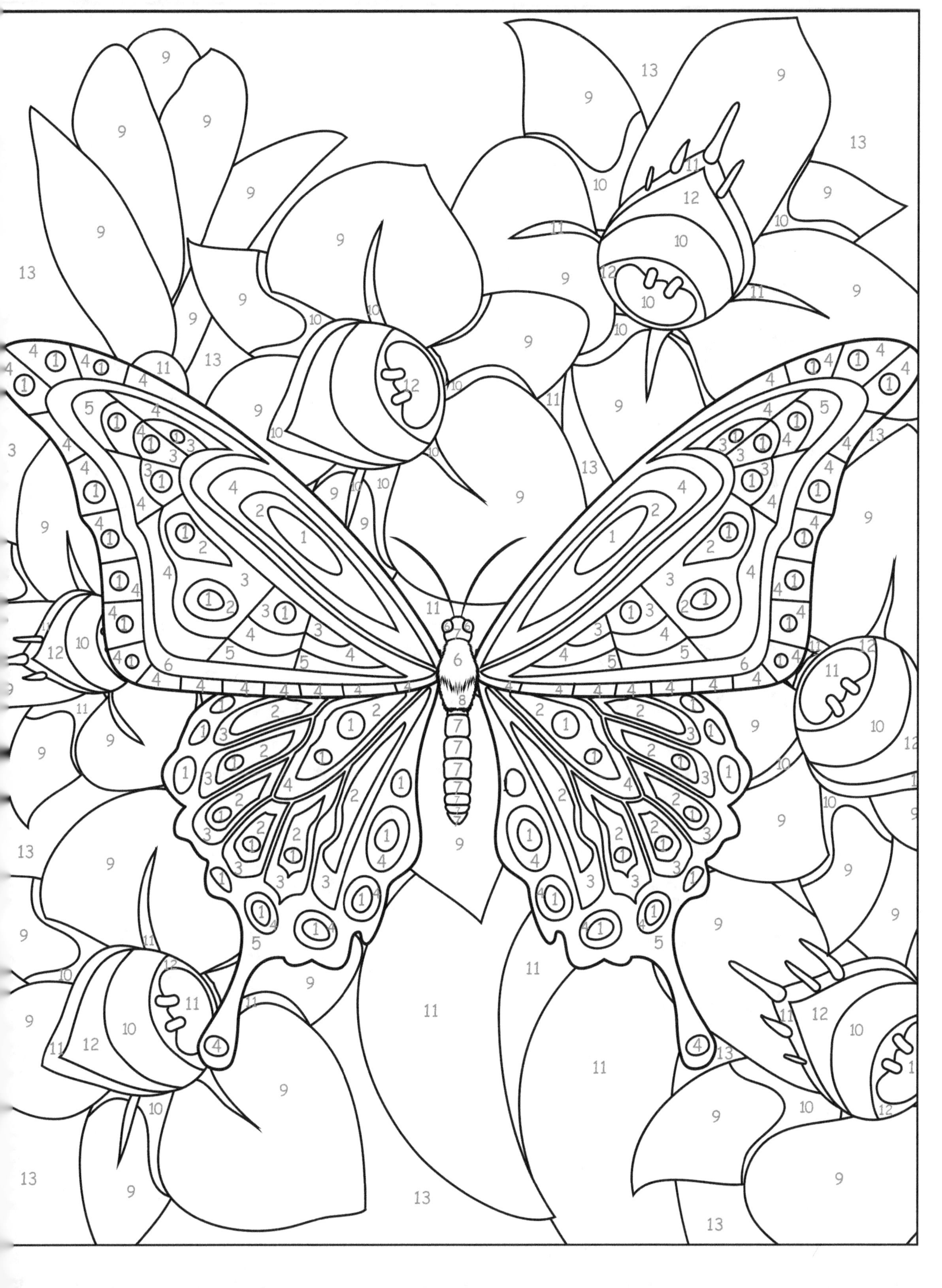

1. Yellow
2. Blue
3. Light Green
4. Orange
5. Magenta
6. Black
7. Dark Purple
8. Brown
9. Green
10. Dark Green
11. Pink
12. Red
13. Cyan
14. Purple

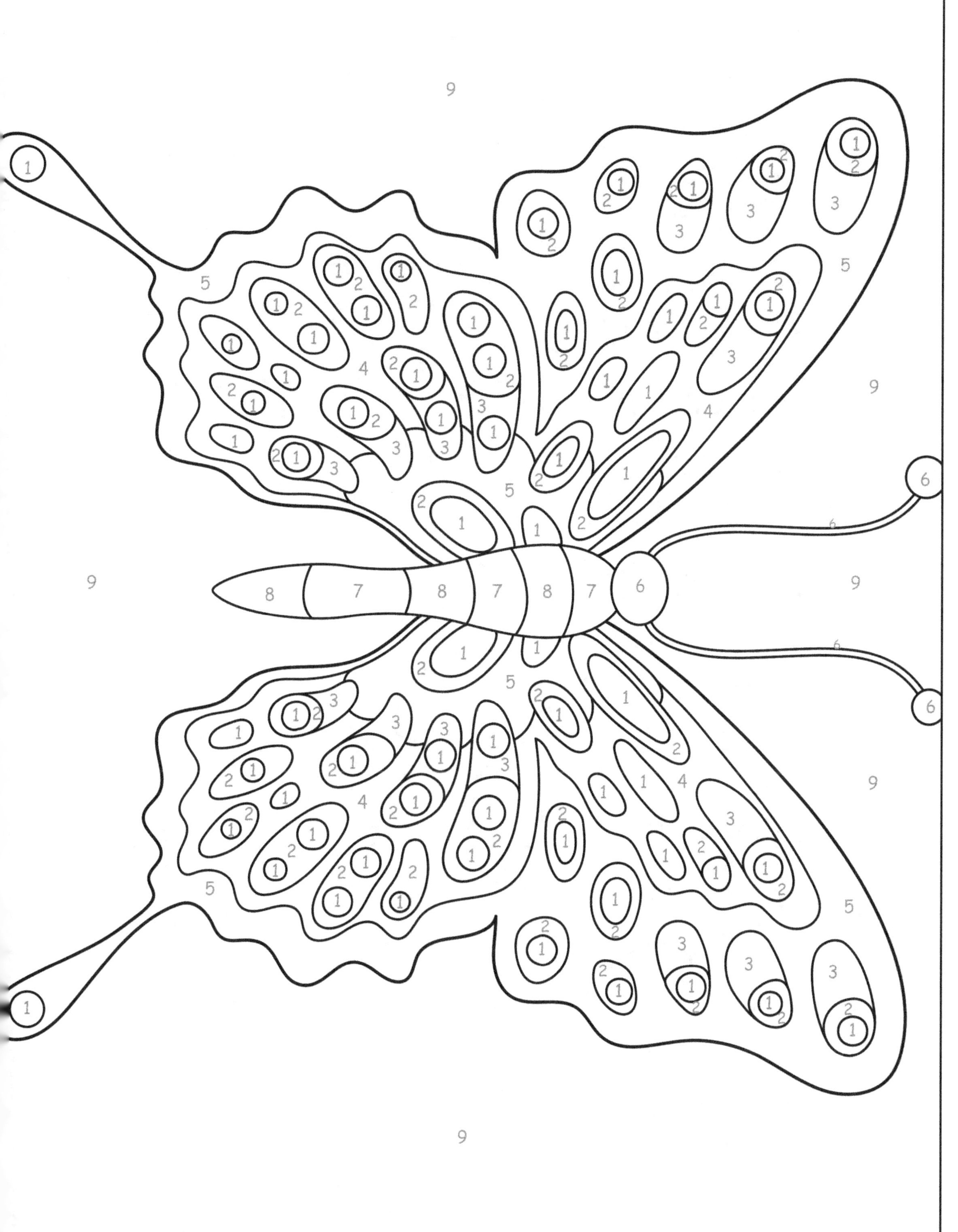

1. Yellow
2. Blue
3. Light Green
4. Orange
5. Magenta
6. Black
7. Dark Purple
8. Brown
9. Green
10. Dark Green
11. Pink
12. Red
13. Cyan
14. Purple

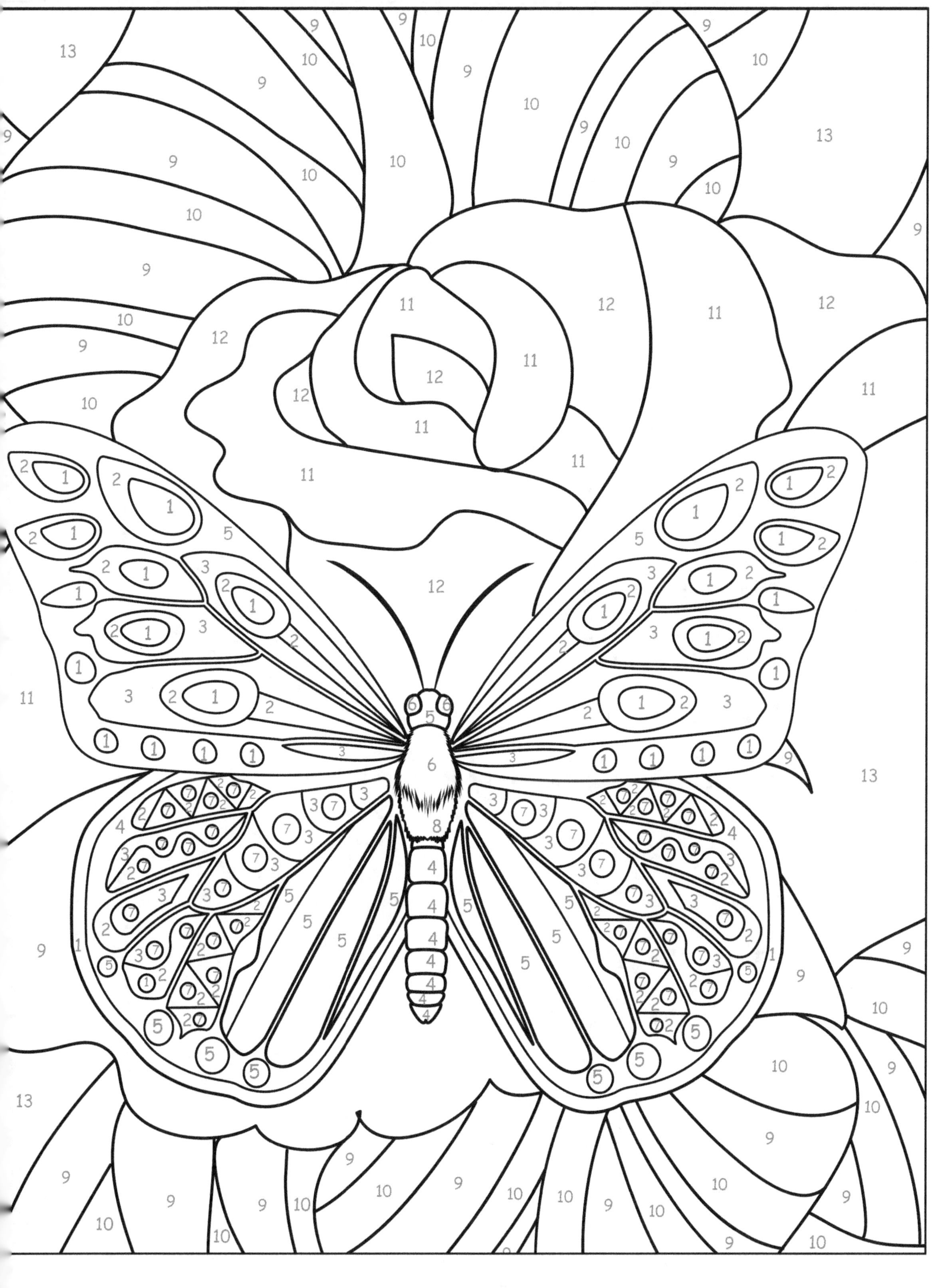

1. Yellow
2. Blue
3. Light Green
4. Orange
5. Magenta
6. Black
7. Dark Purple
8. Brown
9. Green
10. Dark Green
11. Pink
12. Red
13. Cyan
14. Purple

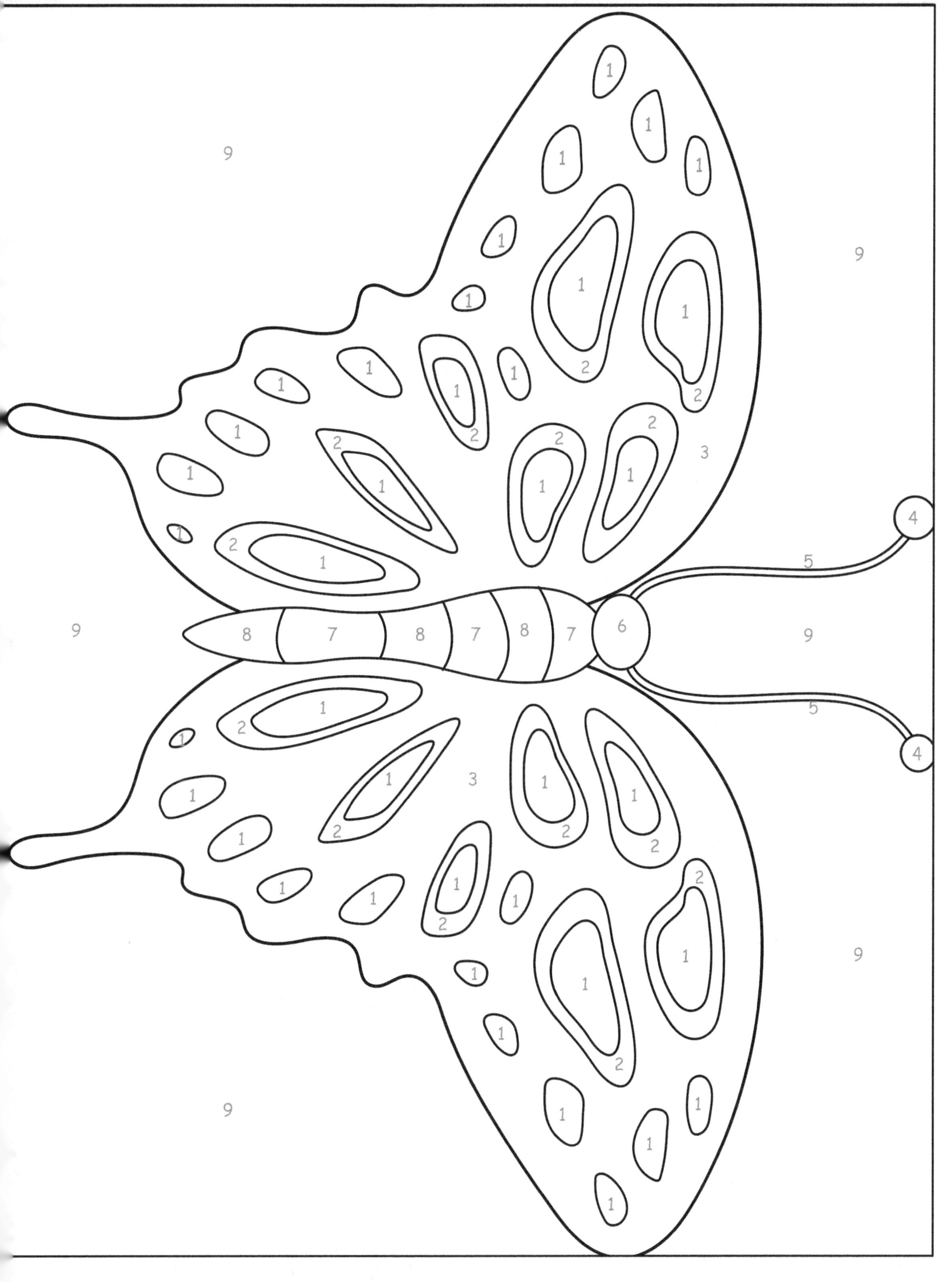

1. Yellow
2. Blue
3. Light Green
4. Orange
5. Magenta
6. Black
7. Dark Purple
8. Brown
9. Green
10. Dark Green
11. Pink
12. Red
13. Cyan
14. Purple

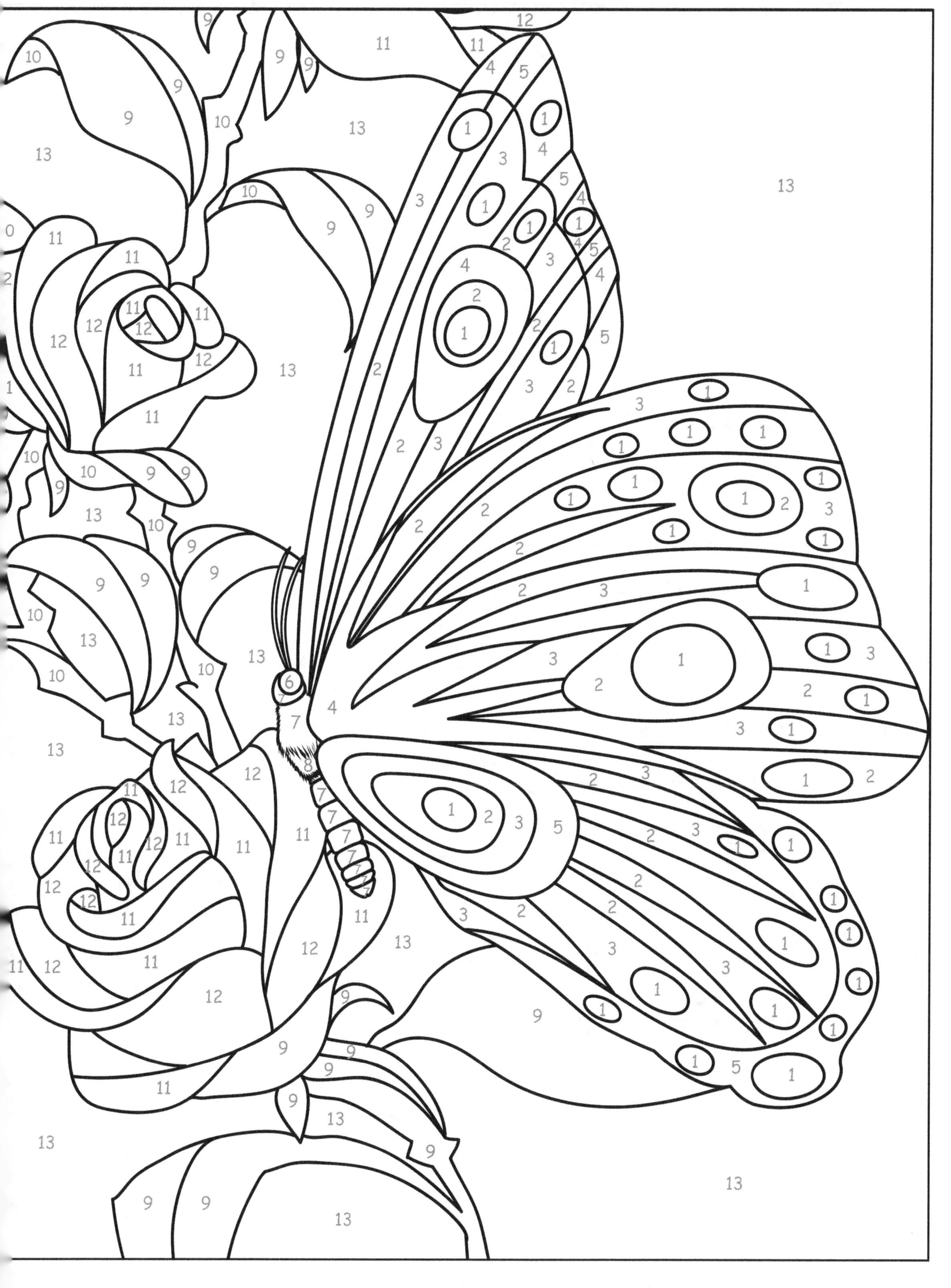

1. Yellow
2. Blue
3. Light Green
4. Orange
5. Magenta
6. Black
7. Dark Purple
8. Brown
9. Green
10. Dark Green
11. Pink
12. Red
13. Cyan
14. Purple

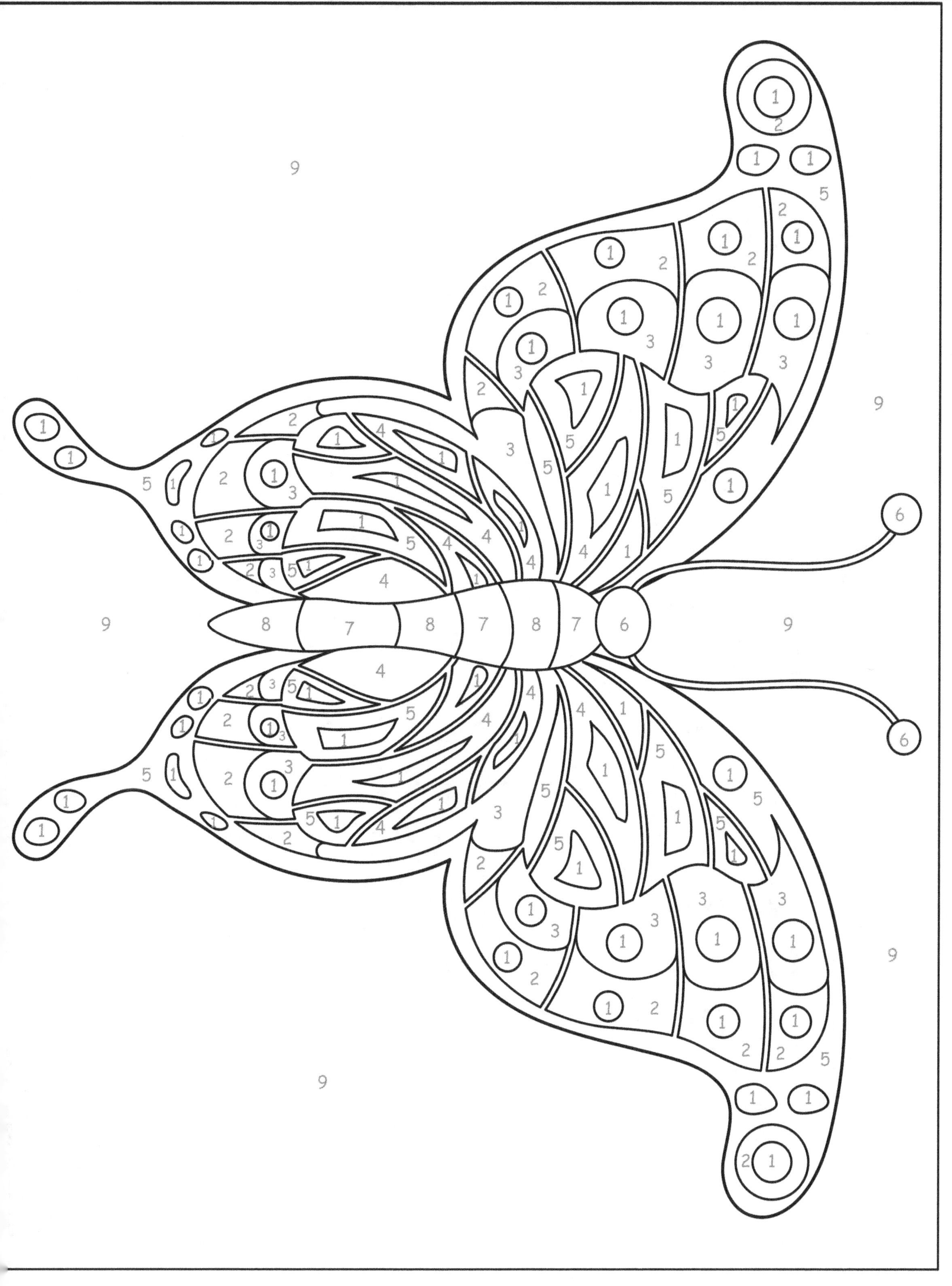

1. Yellow
2. Blue
3. Light Green
4. Orange
5. Magenta
6. Black
7. Dark Purple
8. Brown
9. Green
10. Dark Green
11. Pink
12. Red
13. Cyan
14. Purple

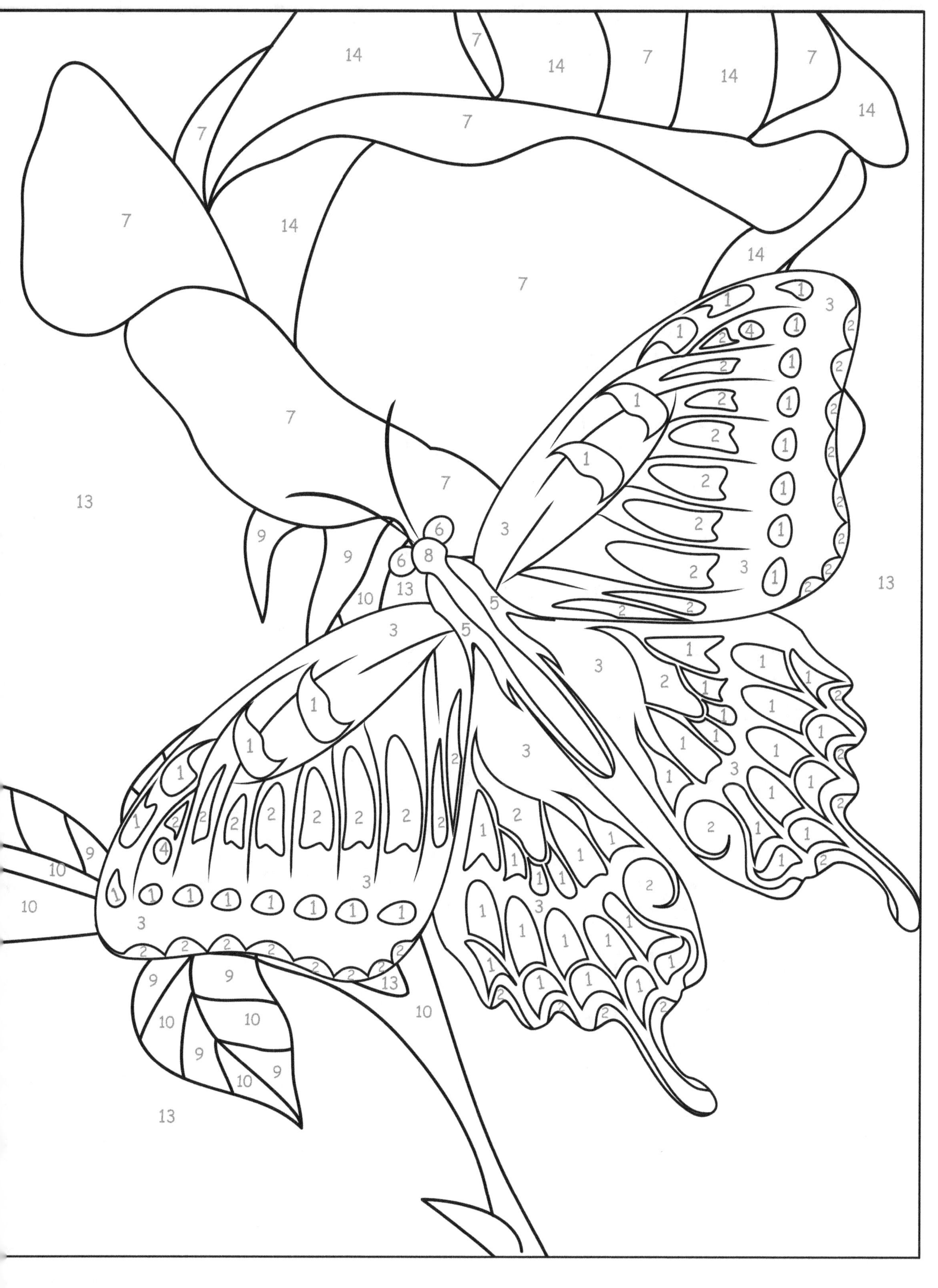

1. Yellow
2. Blue
3. Light Green
4. Orange
5. Magenta
6. Black
7. Dark Purple
8. Brown
9. Green
10. Dark Green
11. Pink
12. Red
13. Cyan
14. Purple

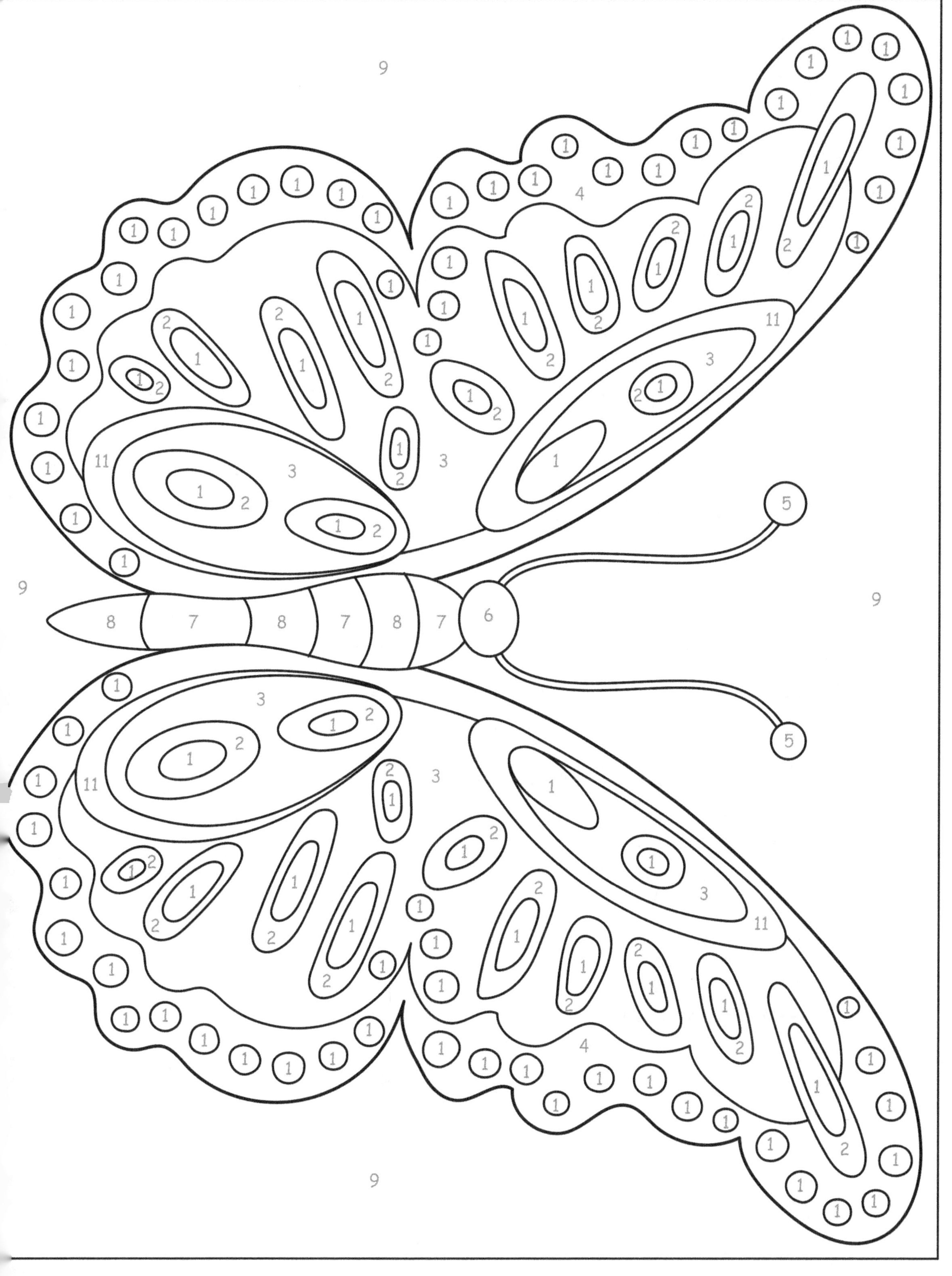

1. Yellow
2. Blue
3. Light Green
4. Orange
5. Magenta
6. Black
7. Dark Purple
8. Brown
9. Green
10. Dark Green
11. Pink
12. Red
13. Cyan
14. Purple

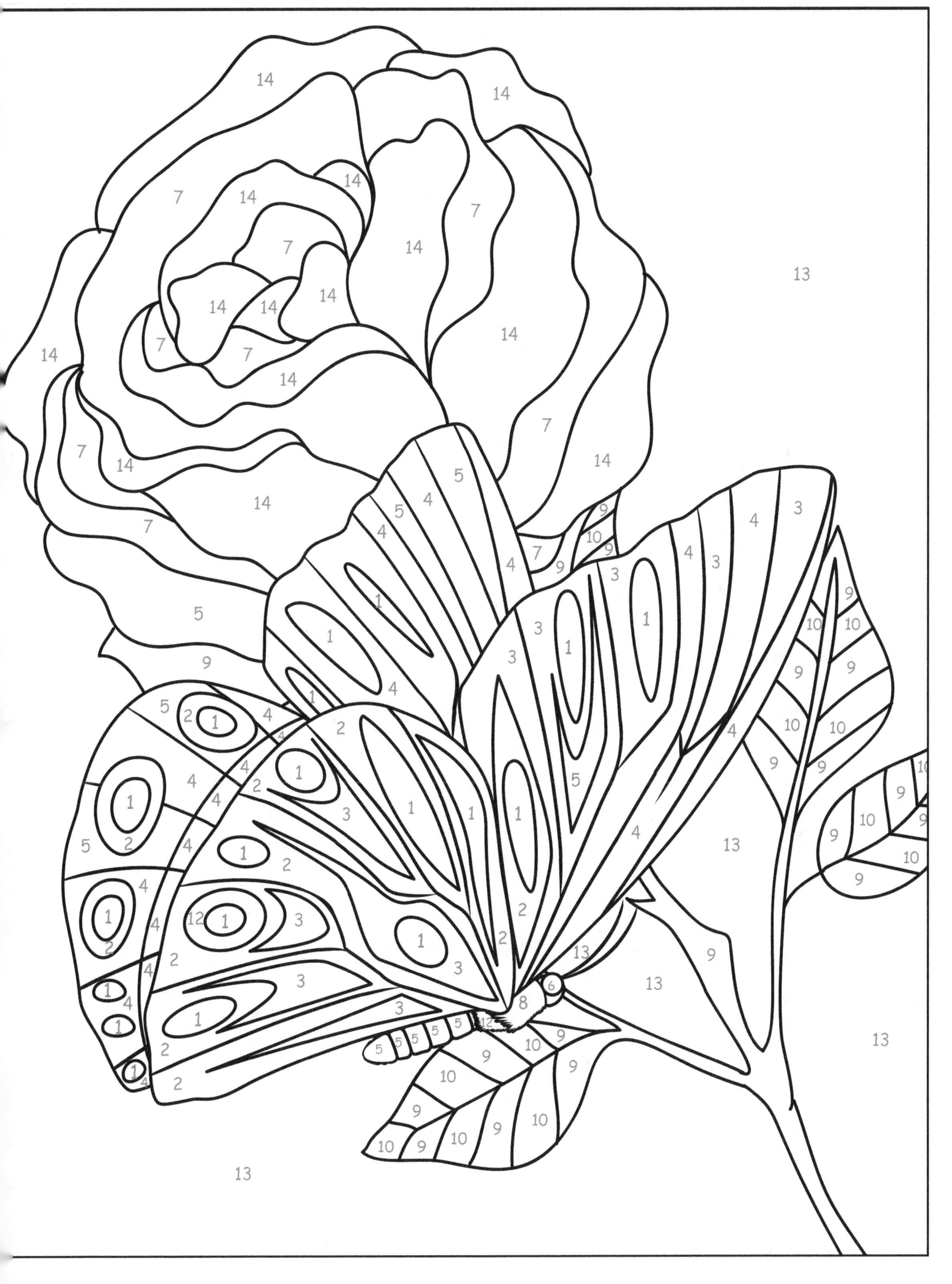

1. Yellow
2. Blue
3. Light Green
4. Orange
5. Magenta
6. Black
7. Dark Purple
8. Brown
9. Green
10. Dark Green
11. Pink
12. Red
13. Cyan
14. Purple

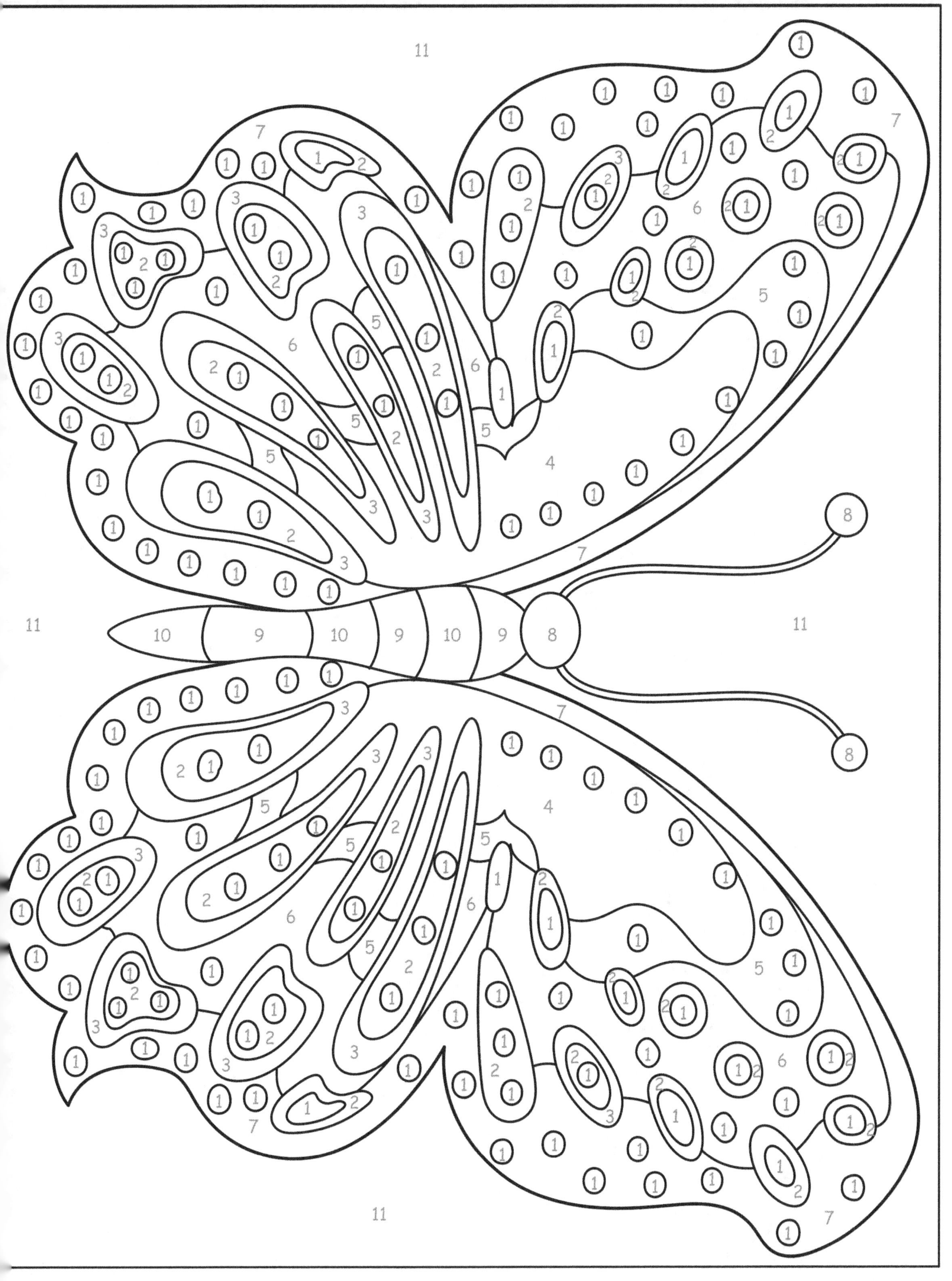

1. Yellow
2. Blue
3. Light Green
4. Orange
5. Magenta
6. Black
7. Dark Purple
8. Brown
9. Green
10. Dark Green
11. Pink
12. Red
13. Cyan
14. Purple

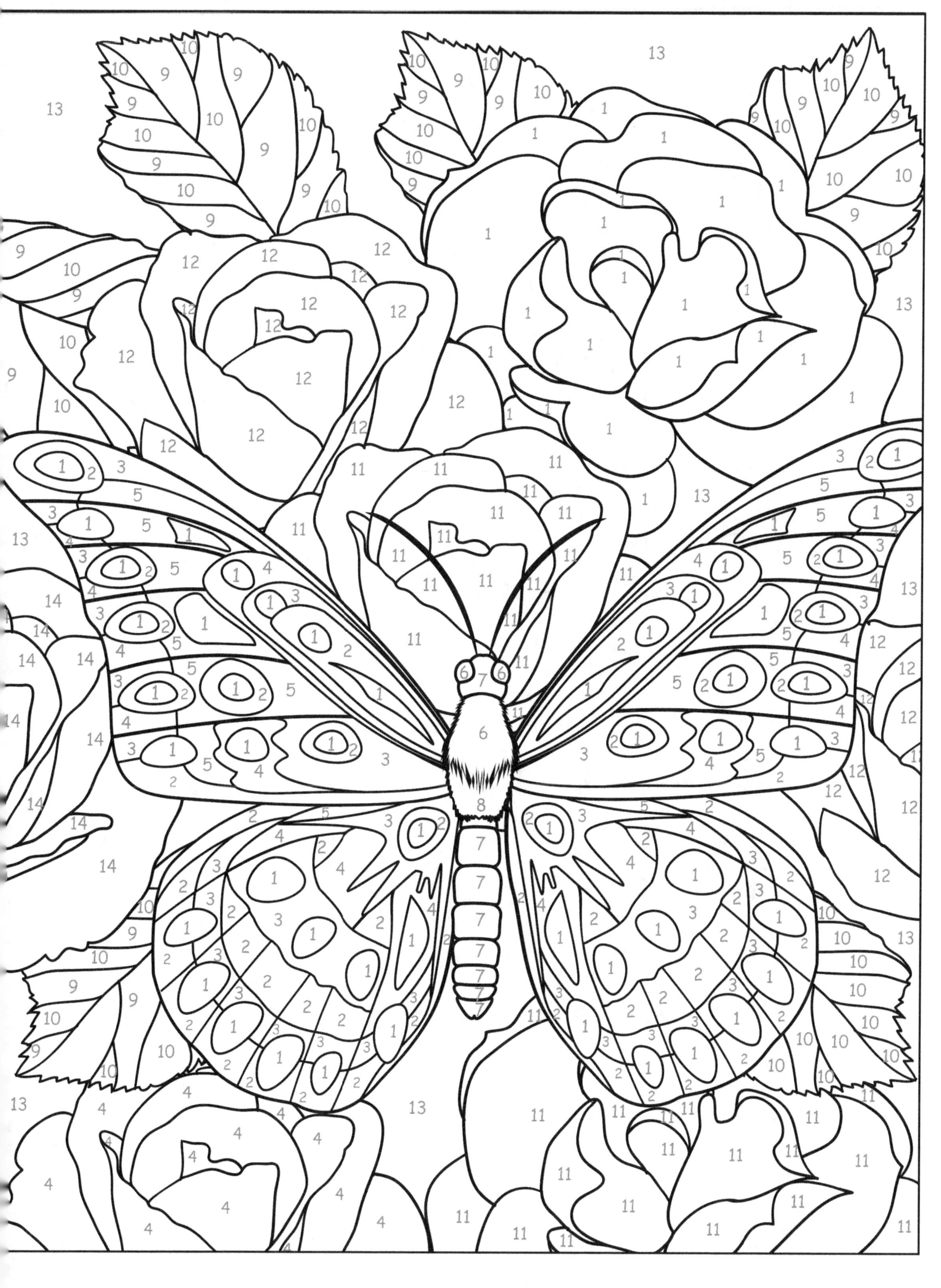

1. Yellow
2. Blue
3. Light Green
4. Orange
5. Magenta
6. Black
7. Dark Purple
8. Brown
9. Green
10. Dark Green
11. Pink
12. Red
13. Cyan
14. Purple

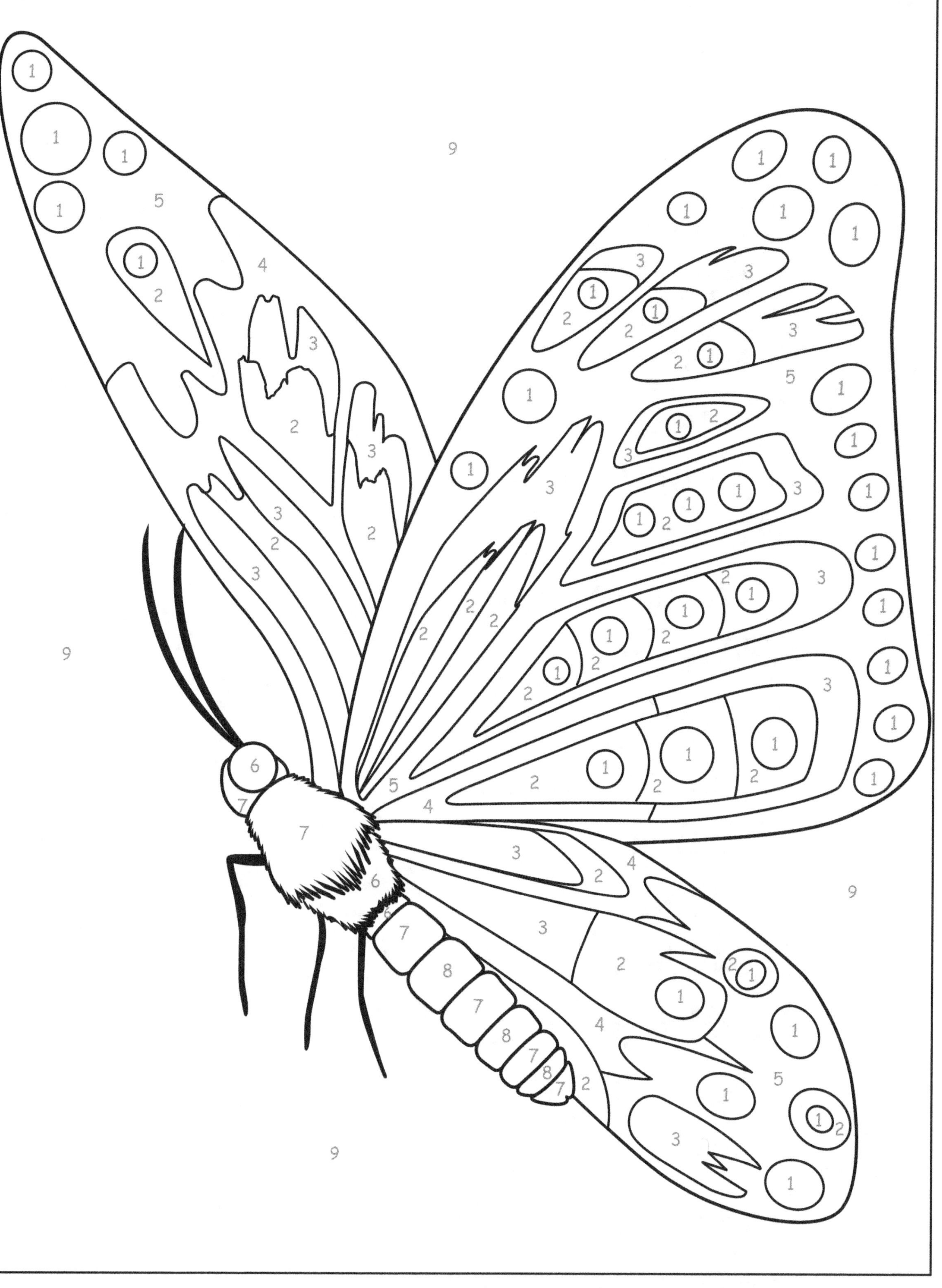

1. Yellow
2. Blue
3. Light Green
4. Orange
5. Magenta
6. Black
7. Dark Purple
8. Brown
9. Green
10. Dark Green
11. Pink
12. Red
13. Cyan
14. Purple

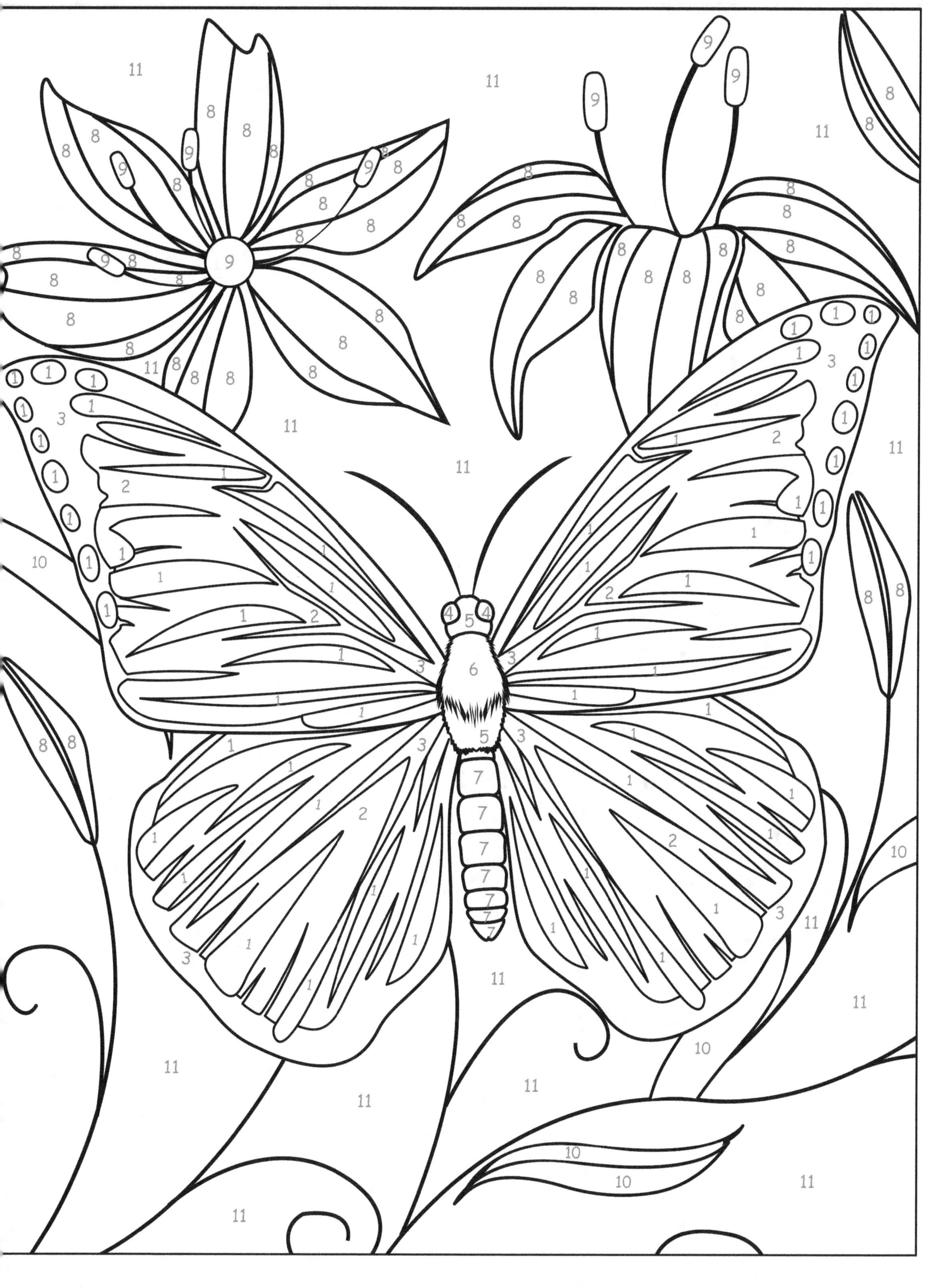

1. Yellow
2. Blue
3. Light Green
4. Orange
5. Magenta
6. Black
7. Dark Purple
8. Brown
9. Green
10. Dark Green
11. Pink
12. Red
13. Cyan
14. Purple

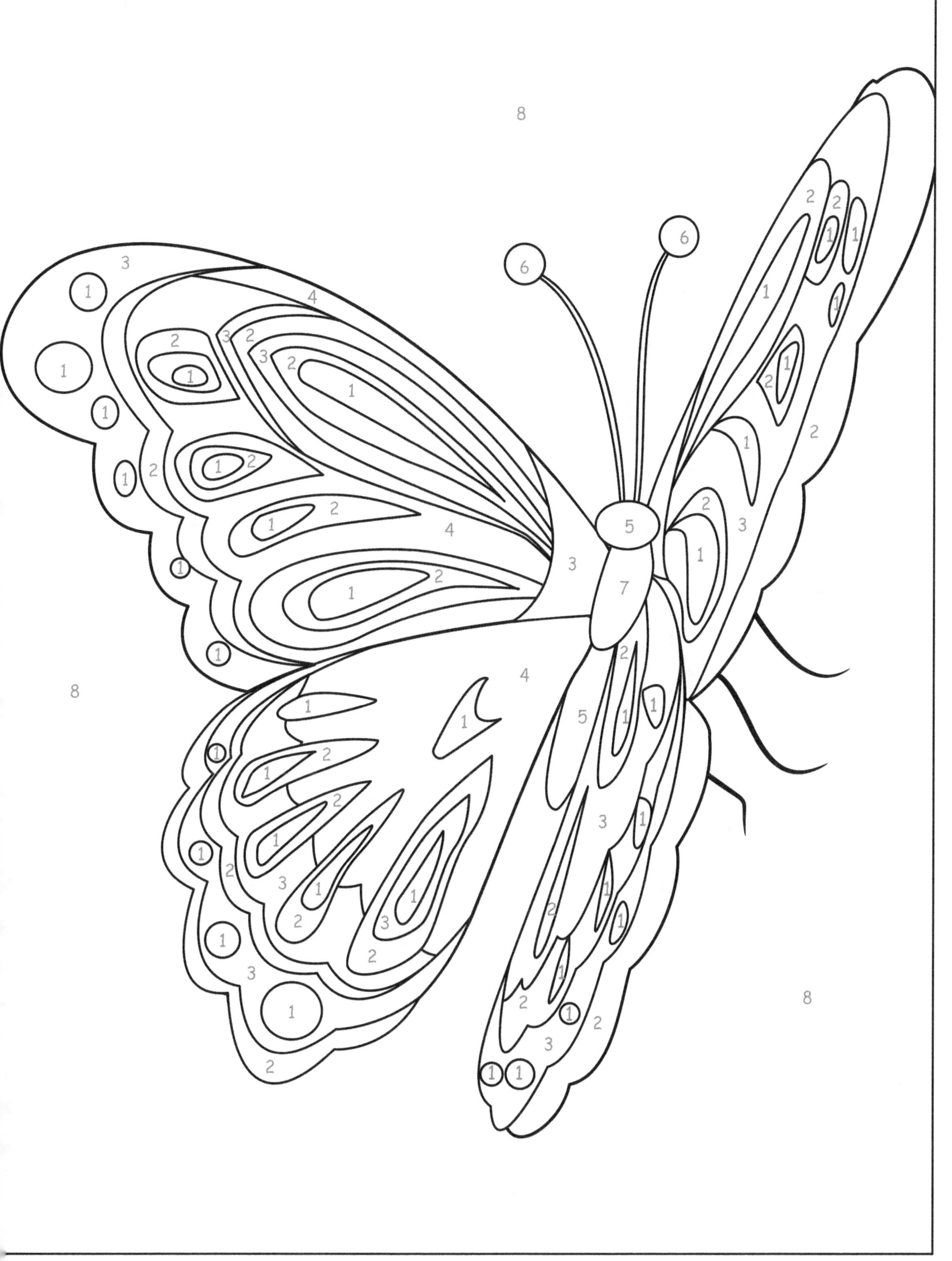

1. Yellow
2. Blue
3. Light Green
4. Orange
5. Magenta
6. Black
7. Dark Purple
8. Brown
9. Green
10. Dark Green
11. Pink
12. Red
13. Cyan
14. Purple

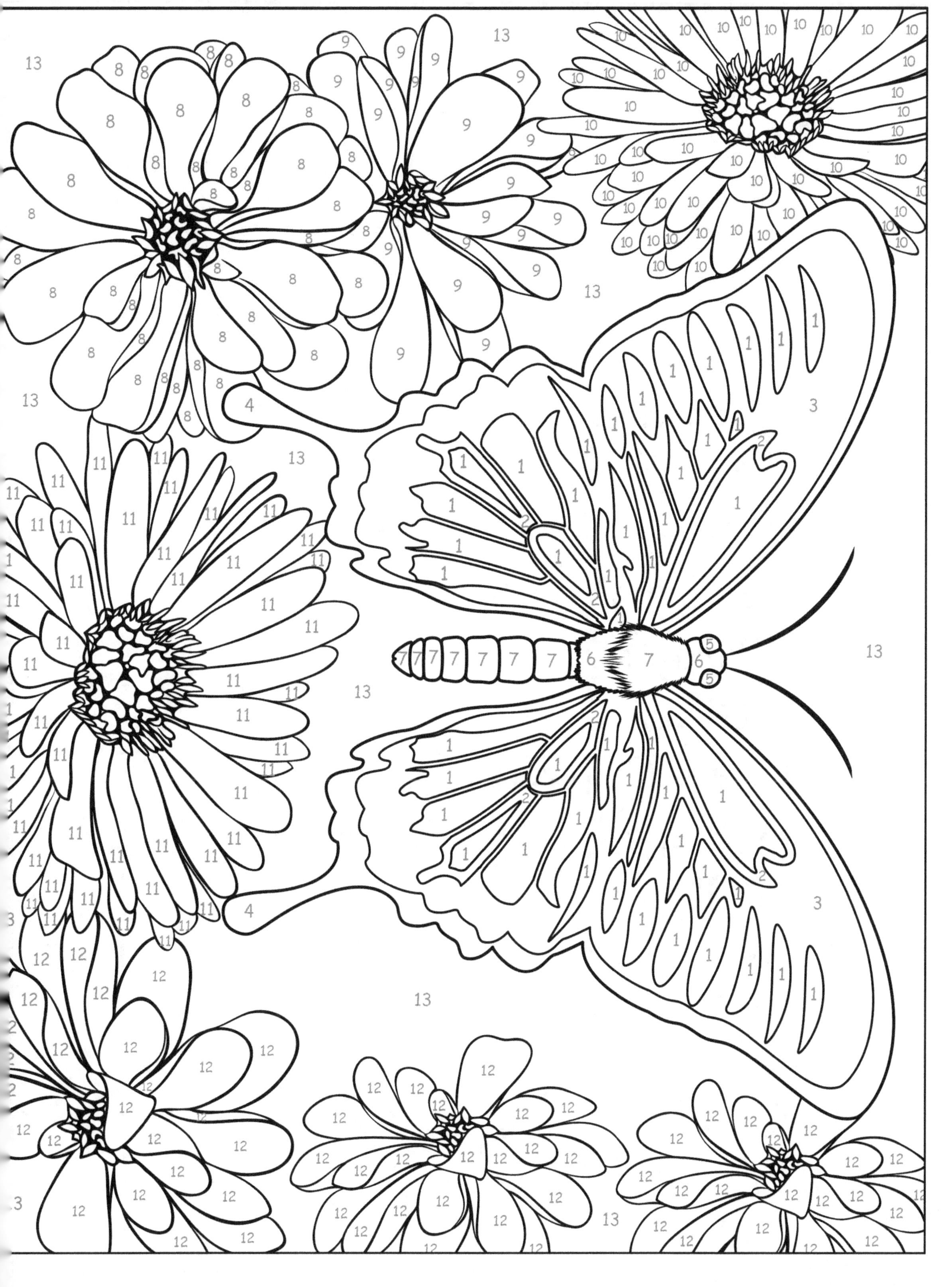

1. Yellow
2. Blue
3. Light Green
4. Orange
5. Magenta
6. Black
7. Dark Purple
8. Brown
9. Green
10. Dark Green
11. Pink
12. Red
13. Cyan
14. Purple

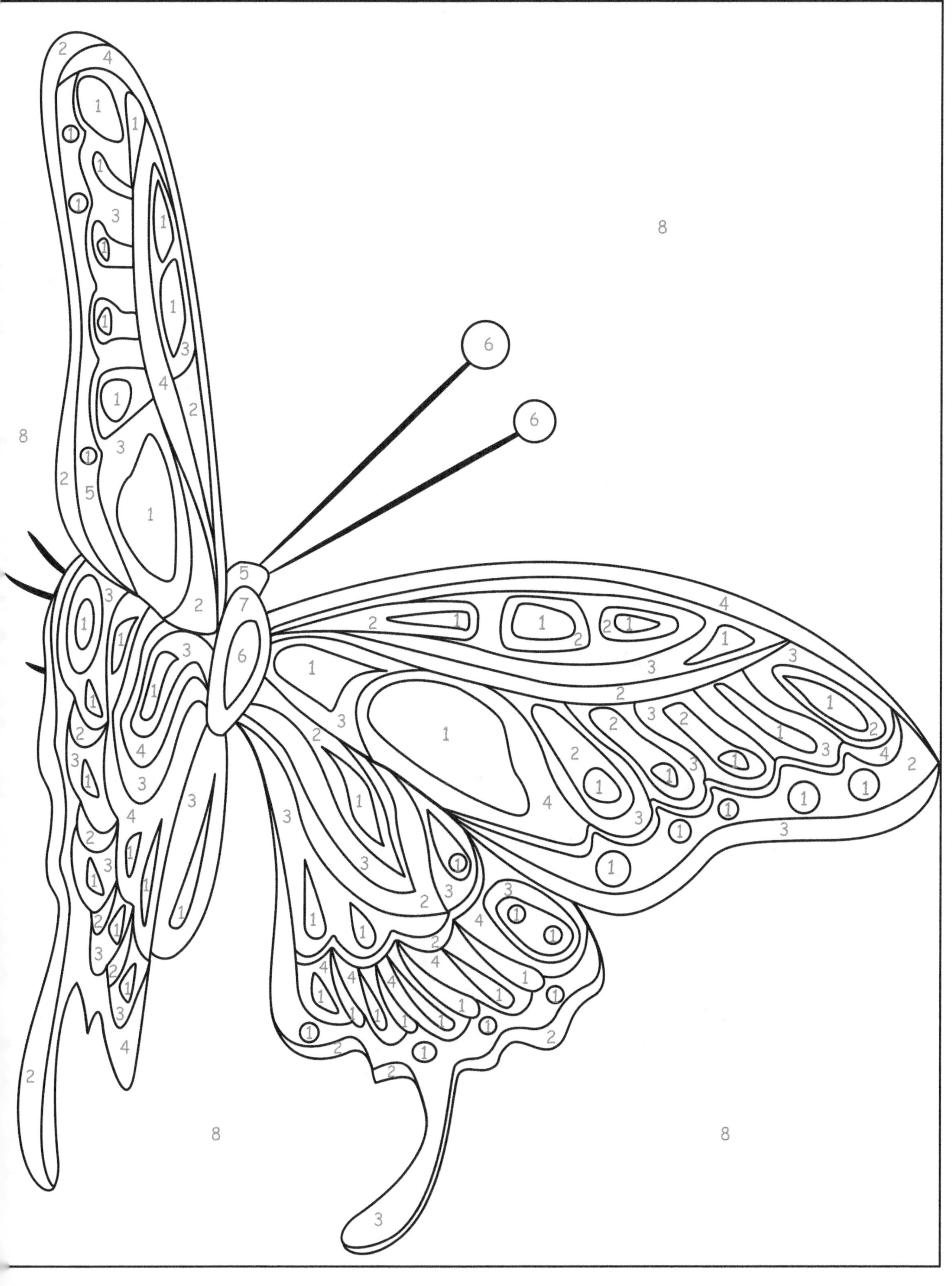

1. Yellow
2. Blue
3. Light Green
4. Orange
5. Magenta
6. Black
7. Dark Purple
8. Brown
9. Green
10. Dark Green
11. Pink
12. Red
13. Cyan
14. Purple

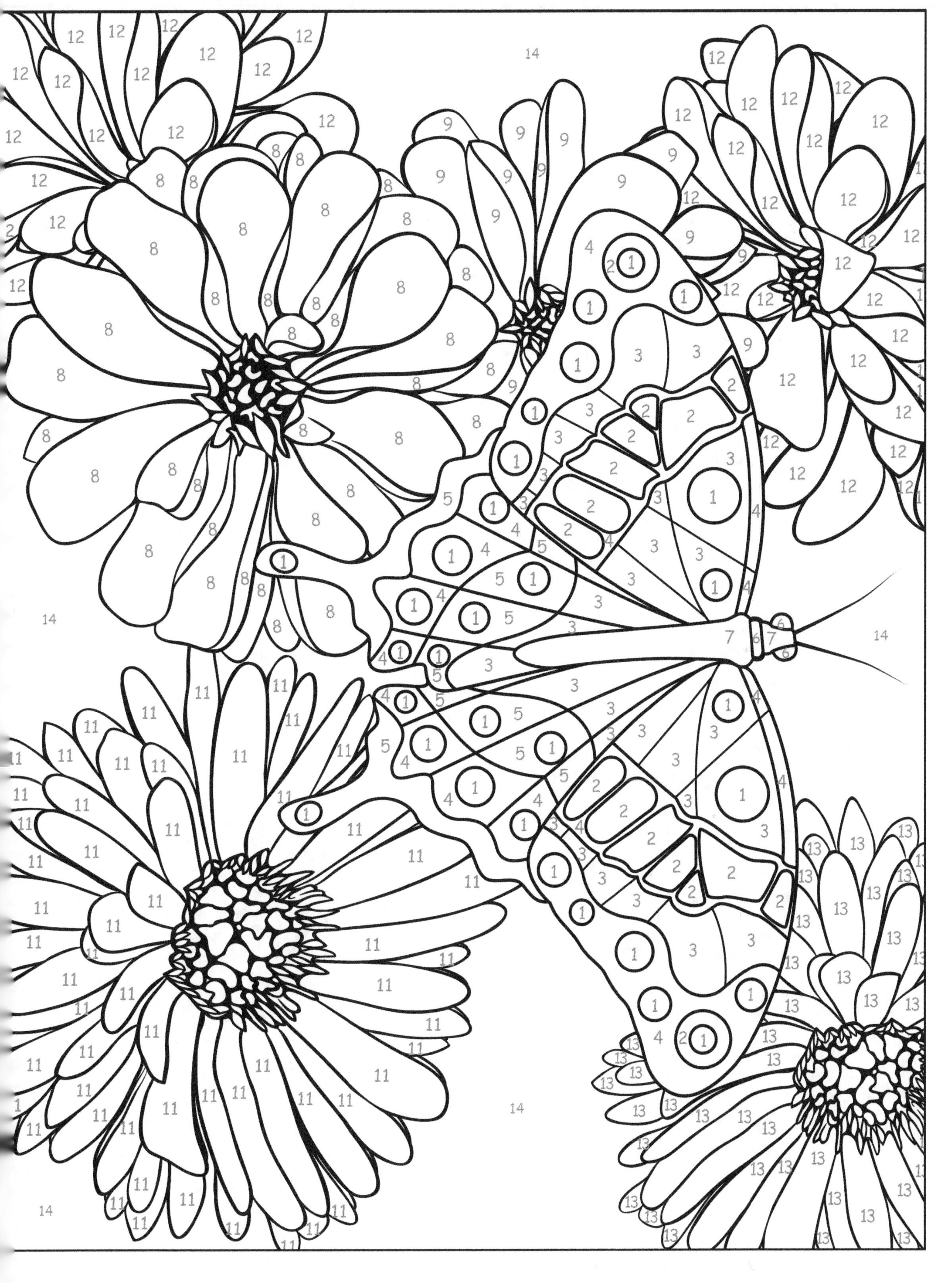

1. Yellow
2. Blue
3. Light Green
4. Orange
5. Magenta
6. Black
7. Dark Purple
8. Brown
9. Green
10. Dark Green
11. Pink
12. Red
13. Cyan
14. Purple

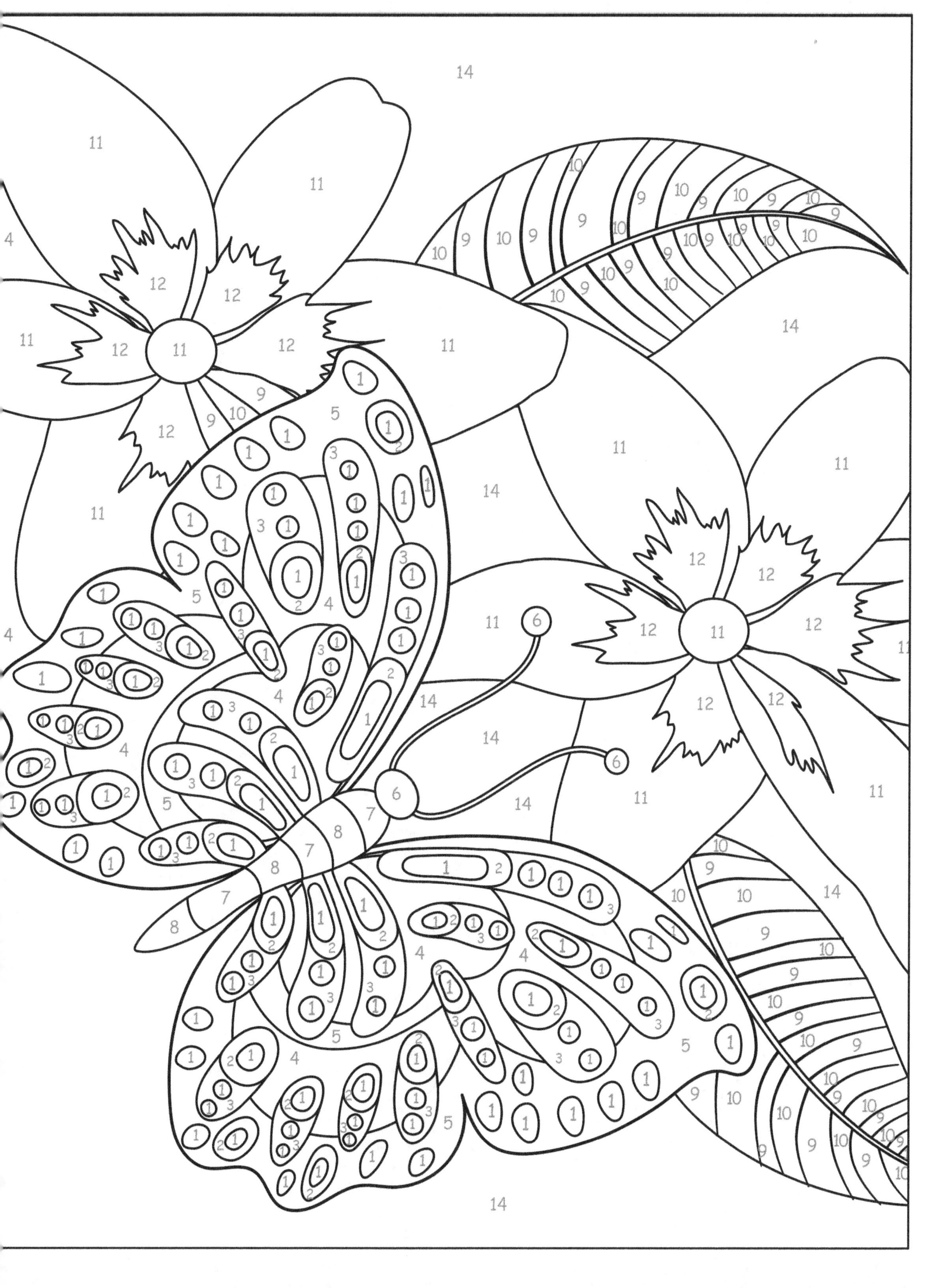

Thank you for supporting
ZenMaster Coloring Books

Your support means the world to us,
and we're thrilled to have you embark on this
creative journey with us.

Our small company strives to make a
BIG difference by helping those
who may be less fortunate.

This is why we proudly hire struggling
artists from around the world!

Our goal is to provide financial support to artists and
their families by enabling them to pursue their passions
and share their hard work and limitless talent with you!

Help support our hard working artists
by leaving a positive review on Amazon!

And follow us on Facebook for updates and
FREE COLORING PAGES!
https://www.facebook.com/zenmastercoloringbooks/

Check out more of our books at:
amazon.com/author/zenmastercoloringbooks

Free Bonus Page!
from:

Large Print Adult Coloring Book of
Mermaids

https://www.amazon.com/dp/1726089274

Also available in color by numbers!!
https://www.amazon.com/dp/1726069745

And 5x8" Travel Size
https://www.amazon.com/dp/1726398315

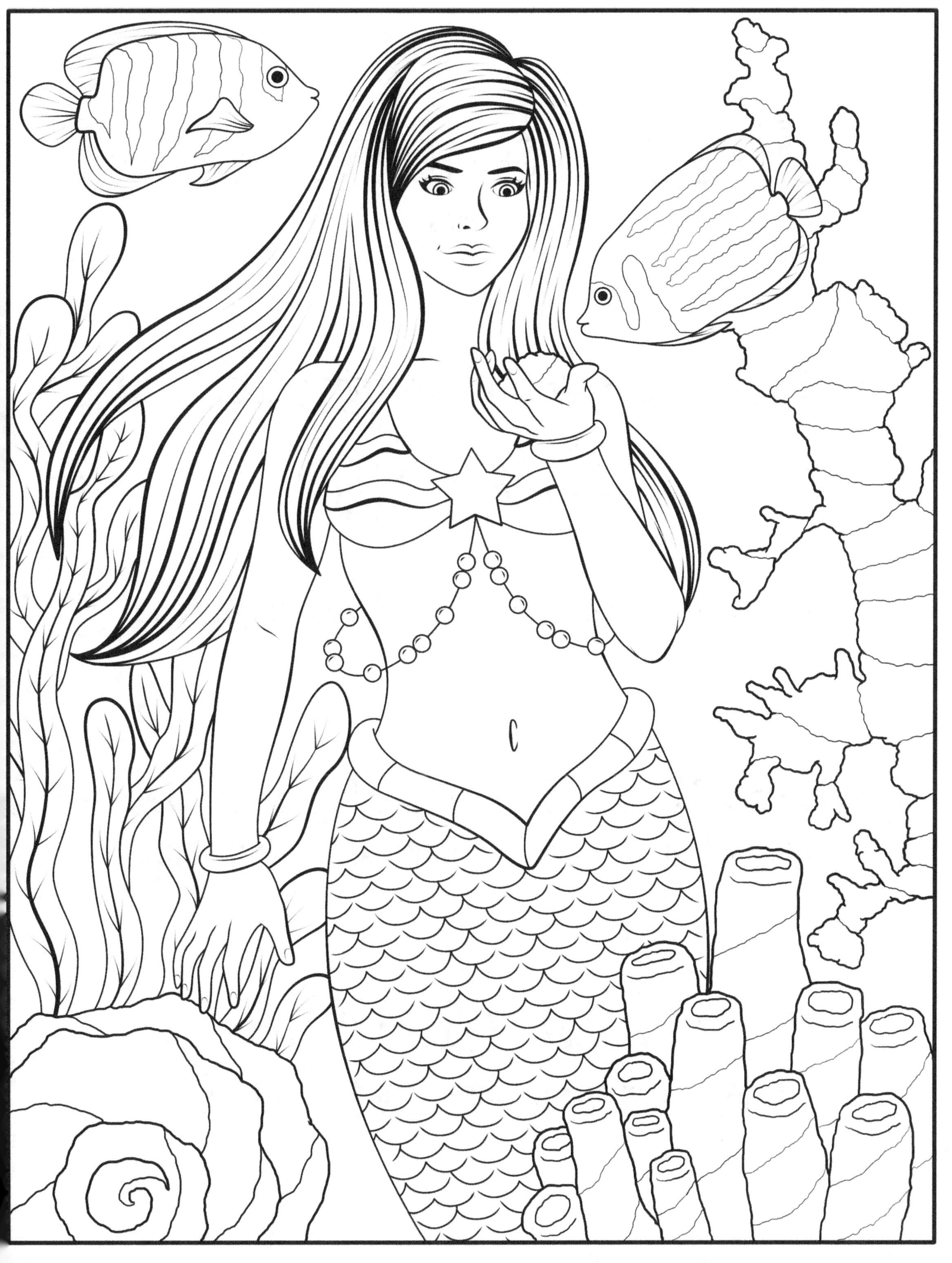

Free Bonus Page!
from:

Large Print Adult Coloring Book of
Spring

https://www.amazon.com/dp/1985347024

Also available in color by numbers!!
https://www.amazon.com/dp/1985375540

And 5x8" Travel Size
https://www.amazon.com/dp/1726193357

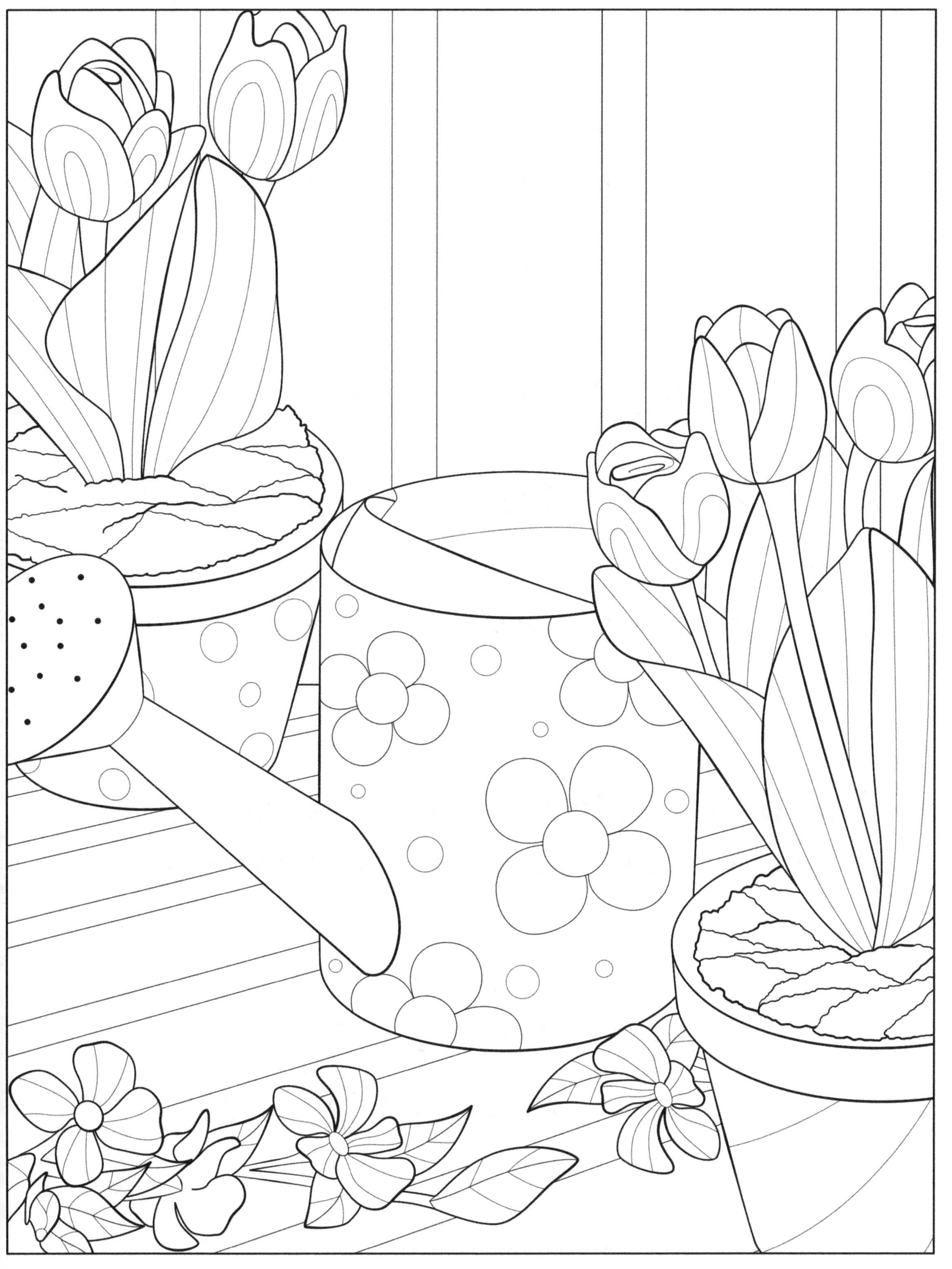

Free Bonus Page!
from:

Adult Coloring Book of
Sweets and Treats

https://www.amazon.com/dp/1795668881

Also available in color by numbers!!
https://www.amazon.com/dp/1795670983

And 5x8" Travel Size
https://www.amazon.com/dp/1796511447

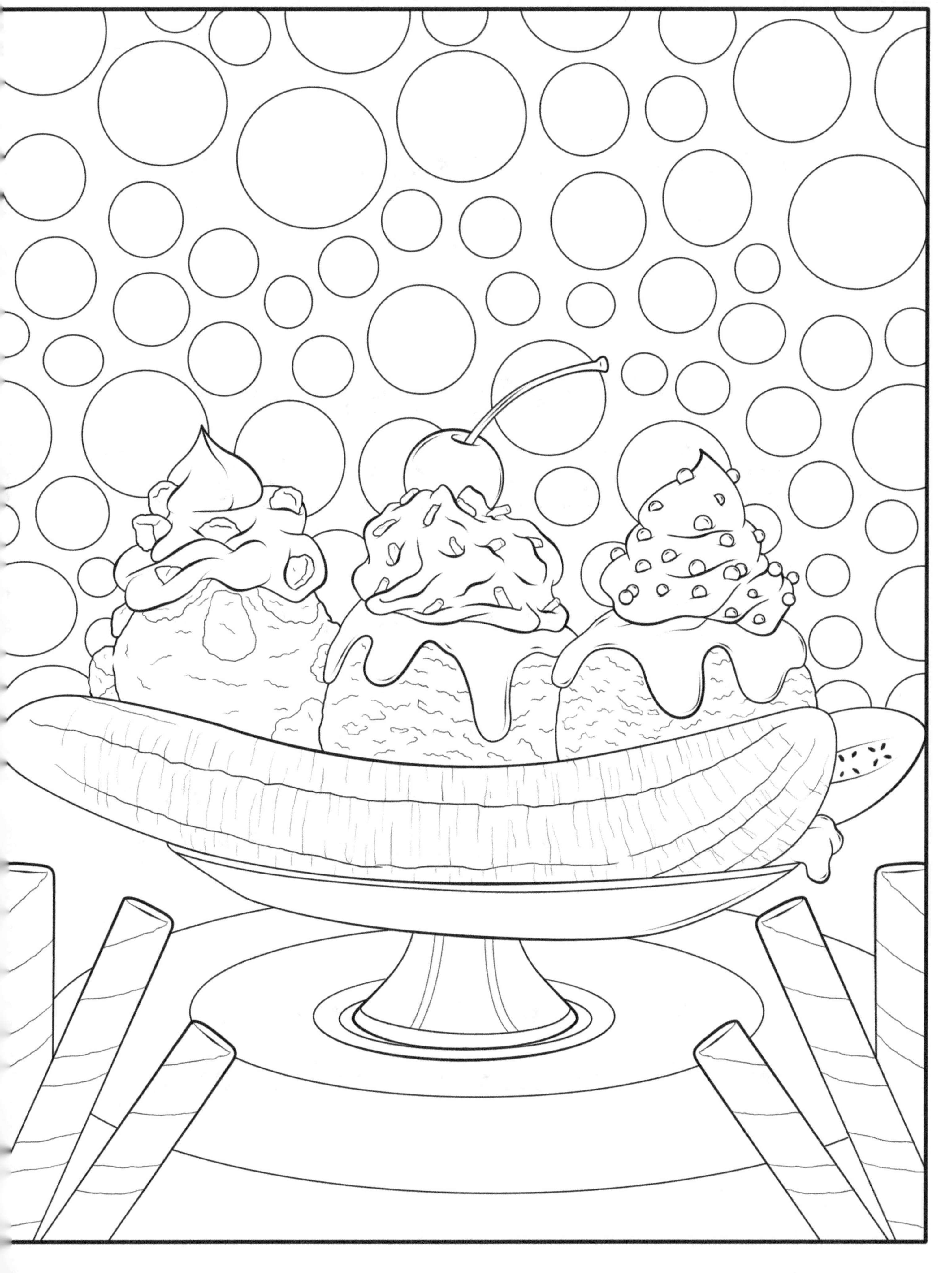

Free Bonus Page!
from:

Adult Coloring Book of
Island Dreams Vacation

https://www.amazon.com/dp/1976291267

Also available in color by numbers!!
https://www.amazon.com/dp/1976507707

And 5x8" Travel Size
https://www.amazon.com/dp/1796516090

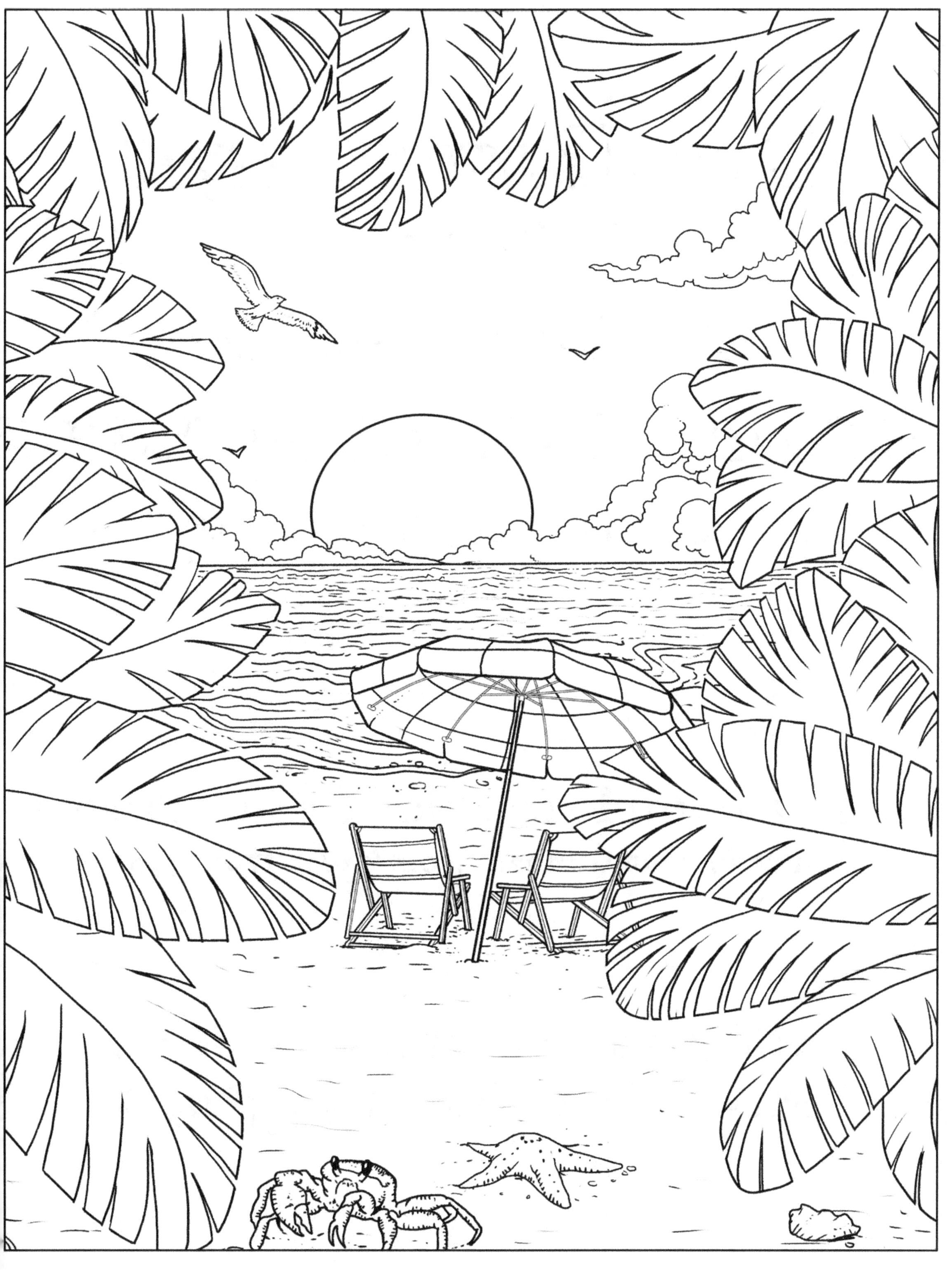

Free Bonus Page!
from:

Extreme dot to dot book of
Butterflies and Flowers

https://amzn.com/dp/1717596746

Also available in color by numbers!!
https://www.amazon.com/dp/1977932398

And a non-numbered edition
https://www.amazon.com/dp/1977882978

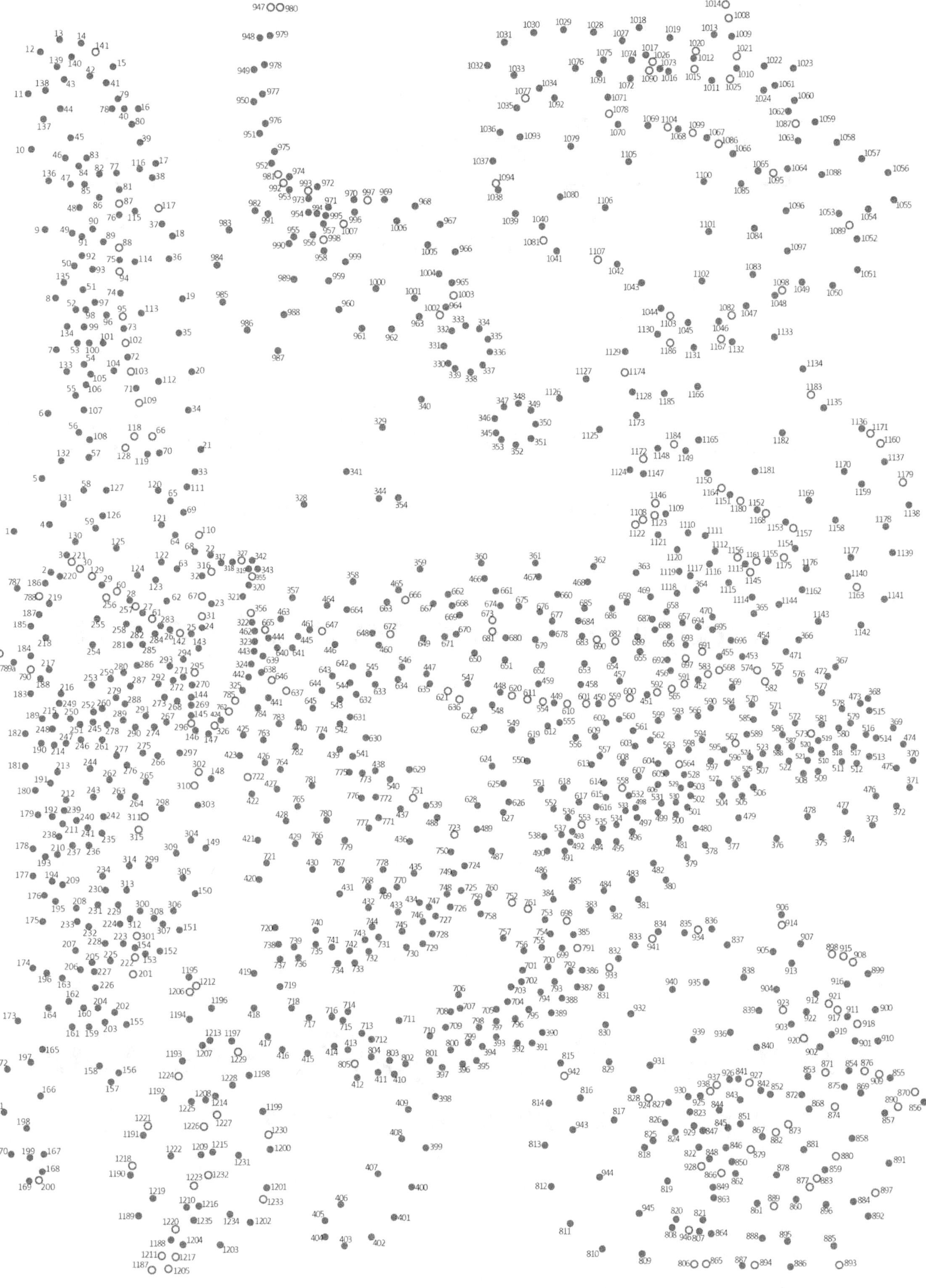

Free Bonus Page!
from:

Zen Coloring Notebook

https://www.amazon.com/dp/1535457015

Available in 9 different colors!

Also available in 5x8" journal size

https://www.amazon.com/dp/1535540591